DIY MEDICAL FACE MASK

CINDY CAPLETON

© Copyright 2020 all right reserved

This document is geared towards providing exact and reliable information about the topic and issue covered. The publication is sold with the idea that the publisher is not required to render accounting, officially permitted or otherwise qualified services. If advice is necessary, legal or professional, a practiced individual in the profession should be ordered. - From a Declaration of Principles which was accepted and approved equally by a Committee of the American Bar Association and a Committee of Publishers and Associations.

In no way is it legal to reproduce, duplicate, or transmit any part of this document in either electronic means or printed format. Recording of this publication is strictly prohibited, and any storage of this document is not allowed unless with written permission from the publisher. All rights reserved. The information provided herein is stated to be truthful and consistent, in that any liability, in terms of inattention or otherwise, by any usage or abuse of any policies, processes, or directions contained within is the sole and utter responsibility of the recipient reader.

Under no circumstances will any legal responsibility or blame be held against the publisher for any reparation, damages, or monetary loss due to the information herein, either directly or indirectly. Respective authors own all copyrights not held by the publisher.

The information herein is offered for informational purposes solely and is universal as so. The presentation of the information is without a contract or any type of guarantee assurance.

TABLE OF CONTENTS

Introduction 1

What You Should Before Making Homemade Face Mask 5

Step By Step Instructions To Wear A Medical Face Mask 17

Steps And Steps Instruction On How To Make Medical Face Mask 30

Types Of Medical Face Mask 36

Benefit Of Medical Face Mask 41

Diy Medical Face Mask Pattern 46

Diy Medical Face Mask Filter 61

Conclusion 72

INTRODUCTION

A boundary gadget utilized in disease control to forestall human services suppliers from breathing or hacking on patients. It is likewise utilized to keep patients' sniffles and sputum from reaching the medicinal services supplier's face or eyes or from being breathed in.

A gadget that covers the mouth, nose, or both of a patient who requires positive-pressure, noninvasive ventilation or nonstop positive weight ventilation (CPAP).

A careful mask, otherwise called a methodology mask, medical mask or just as a face mask, is proposed to be worn by wellbeing experts during medical procedure and during nursing to get the microbes shed in fluid beads and pressurized canned products from the wearer's mouth and nose. They are intended to shield the wearer from breathing in airborne microorganisms or infection particles, however are less viable than respirators, for example, N95 or FFP masks, which give better insurance because of their material, shape and tight seal.

Careful masks fluctuate by quality and levels of insurance. In spite of their name, not every single careful mask are proper to be utilized during medical procedures. Careful masks might be named as careful, disconnection, dental, or medical strategy masks. Chinese wellbeing authorities recognize medical (non-careful) and careful masks.

Careful masks are made of a nonwoven texture made utilizing a soften blowing process. They came into utilization during the 1960s and generally supplanted fabric facemasks in created nations. The utilization of careful masks during the continuous 2019–20 coronavirus pandemic has been a subject of discussion, as deficiencies of careful masks is a focal issue.

Careful masks are prevalently worn by the overall population lasting through the year in East Asian nations like China, Japan and South Korea to lessen the opportunity of spreading airborne ailments to other people, and to forestall the taking in of airborne residue particles made via air contamination. Furthermore, careful masks have become a design proclamation, especially in contemporary East Asian culture reinforced by its fame in Japanese and Korean mainstream society which bigly affect East Asian youth culture.

The structure of the careful masks relies upon the mode; ordinarily, the masks are three-employ (three layers). This three-employ material is comprised of a liquefy blown polymer, most usually polypropylene, set between non-woven texture. The liquefy blown material goes about as the channel that prevents organisms from entering or leaving the mask. Creases are generally used to permit the client to grow the mask to such an extent that it covers the region from the nose to the jawline. The masks are made sure about to the head with ear circles, head ties, or flexible lashes.

A careful mask, or strategy mask, is expected to be worn by wellbeing experts during medical procedure and certain medicinal services methodology to get microorganisms shed in fluid beads and pressurized canned products from the wearer's mouth and nose.

Proof backings the viability of careful masks in diminishing the danger of contamination among other human services laborers and in the network. In any case, a Cochrane survey found that there is no reasonable proof that expendable face masks worn by individuals from the careful group would lessen the danger of twisted diseases after clean careful procedures.

For human services laborers, wellbeing rules suggest the wearing of a face-fit tried N95 or FFP3 respirator mask rather than a careful mask in the region of pandemic-influenza patients, to diminish the presentation of the wearer to conceivably irresistible pressurized canned products and airborne fluid beads.

WHAT YOU SHOULD BEFORE MAKING HOMEMADE FACE MASK

──────── ♦◇♦ ────────

Referring to new information that a "significant bit" of individuals contaminated with the novel coronavirus can spread the infection to others in any event, when they don't have indications, the Centers for Disease Control and Prevention updated its proposal, saying that individuals should wear fabric face covers "at whatever point individuals must go into open settings."

A fabric face covering isn't expected to ensure the wearer, yet may keep the spread of infection from the wearer to other people. "This would be particularly significant if somebody is contaminated yet doesn't have manifestations."

On April 3, the Centers for Disease Control and Prevention (CDC) declared new rules suggesting that everybody wear face masks in open settings, regardless of whether they don't feel wiped out, to abstain from spreading the novel coronavirus. The CDC asks that careful and respirator (N95) masks be put something aside for medical staff, such a large number of individuals are making their own. If you're going to attempt to DIY—out of a bandanna, scarf, or other texture you have lying around—this is what you have to think about what accomplishes and doesn't work.

For what reason do I have to wear a mask?

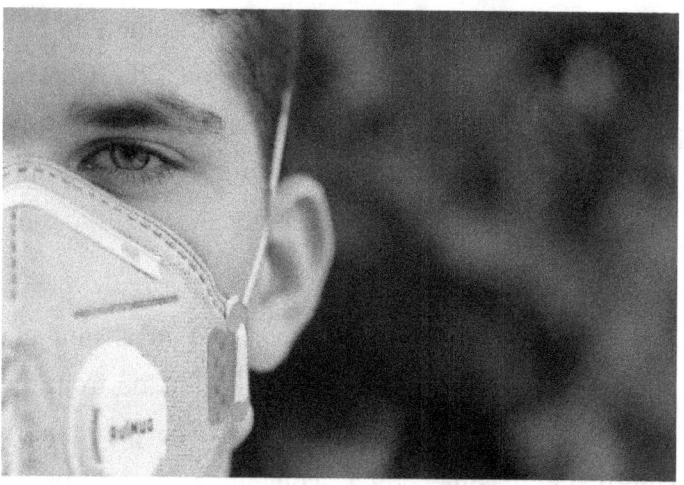

In spite of the fact that specialists said that mask-wearing was superfluous from the outset, the CDC has as of late changed its intuition regarding the matter. New research proposes that not exclusively could an individual unconsciously convey the infection for a normal of four to five days before creating indications, yet numerous individuals with the infection could likewise be asymptomatic, demonstrating no side effects by any means. In the two cases, these individuals are as yet infectious. While wearing a mask doesn't ensure that you won't become ill, it does significantly bring down the danger of pre-symptomatic or asymptomatic individuals spreading the infection to other people, as per the CDC.

When would it be a good idea for me to wear a mask?

The CDC suggests wearing a material face mask whenever you have to leave your home. That incorporates setting off to the supermarket, getting takeout nourishment, and in any event, going on open air runs or strolls. Yet, covering your face with a hand crafted mask doesn't mean you can loosen up other social separating measures. Face masks ought to give extra insurance to basic trips where you can't generally remain six feet from others—yet you should even now stay away from huge, discretionary parties, the CDC says.

What material would it be a good idea for me to utilize?

Not all face masks are made equivalent, and some are increasingly successful at shielding you from approaching germs than others. Research demonstrates that the best material to use for face masks is unified with a thick, tight weave, which squares progressively popular particles from going through. In the wake of testing masks made with a wide range of textures, analysts at the Wake Forest Institute for Regenerative Medicine found that the best masks were made with a heavyweight "quilter's cotton," which has a string tally of in any event 180.

No quilter's cotton? Forget about it. Pillowcases with 600-string check, thick wool night robe, and even vacuum cleaner sacks are likewise affirmed other options, as long as it's layered and you can inhale serenely. If you don't have the foggiest idea what texture to utilize, specialists recommend one basic dependable guideline: "Hold it up to a brilliant light," Dr. Scott Segal, director of anesthesiology at Wake Forest Baptist Health, told the New York Times. "If light goes actually effectively through the strands and you can nearly observe the filaments, it is anything but a decent texture. If it's a denser weave of thicker material and light doesn't go through it so much, that is the material you need to utilize."

Scarves and cotton bandannas, then again, are among the least viable mask-production materials, as indicated by an ongoing report at the Missouri University of Science and Technology. In any case, the researchers found that bandanna masks furnish more filtration when layered with a couple of espresso channels. Fret don't as well if you don't have the ideal material; simply work with what you have. All in all, examines show that any face covering is better than nothing for easing back the spread of coronavirus.

Do I have to realize how to sew?

No. If you have an old T-shirt and some scissors lying around, you're good to go. The CDC has posted two patterns for DIY face masks on its site, including a no-sew alternative. Top health spokesperson Jerome Adams likewise discharged a video telling the best way to a mask out of fabric and elastic groups—no needle and string required.

For what reason wouldn't i be able to wear a careful or respirator mask?

Medical-grade masks, as N95 and careful masks, offer incredible assurance against COVID-19. In any case, these masks are hard to come by. The CDC has mentioned we spare medical-grade masks for medicinal services laborers, who are presented to an a lot higher portion of COVID-19 regularly than the normal individual. These masks ought to likewise be held for high-hazard people, who are more in danger of creating serious complexities from the infection.

Have confidence that custom made face masks made with thick material are about as compelling as medical-grade masks, particularly if you are simply making a speedy excursion to the market. In the Missouri University study, two layers of a sensitivity decrease HVAC channel caught 94 percent of airborne particles, six layers of heater channels caught 95 percent, and four layers of high-string check pillowcases caught almost 60 percent. (Make a point to put the channels between two bits of material texture to abstain from breathing in any hurtful strands.) By examination, careful masks sift through 62 to 65 percent of particles and N95 masks sift through 95 percent of particles. The primary concern: N95 masks are one of the coronavirus items you shouldn't squander your cash on.

In what manner should the mask fit?

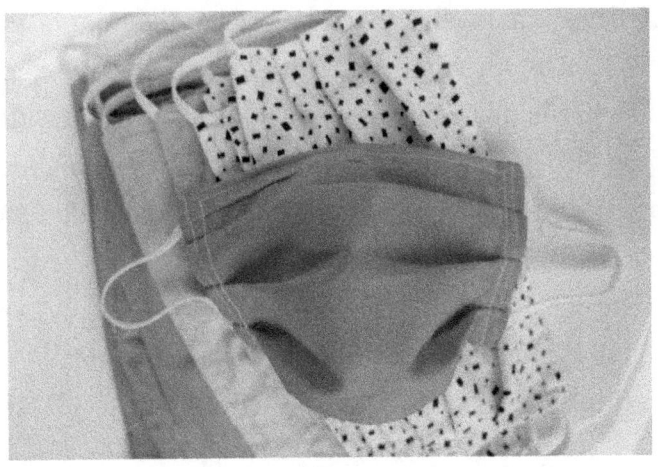

Your mask should fit cozily from the extension of your nose to underneath your jawline, as indicated by the CDC rules. Secure the mask with circles or ties and fix them until the mask fits serenely around your face without holes. Attempt to fight the temptation to alter it while out in the open, which would lead you to contact your face and hazard spreading germs from your hands. Face mask or not, washing your hands consistently and effectively can forestall coronavirus and a not insignificant rundown of different illnesses.

How would I take the mask on and off?

Above all else, you ought to consistently wash your hands when wearing a face mask, specialists state. To take the mask on and off your face, snatch the ties or circles around your ears as opposed to the front of the mask. Abstain from contacting your eyes, nose, or mouth simultaneously, too. For the mask to be the best, the CDC suggests putting it on and expelling it at home, just as saving it in position for the whole time you are out in broad daylight.

In what manner would it be advisable for me to think about my mask?

So as to keep the infection under control, it's basic to clean your masks consistently. A cycle in the clothes washer with high temp water and cleanser will carry out the responsibility, the CDC says. Fabric masks ought to be washed in water that is at any rate 167 degrees F (75 degrees C), the base temperature appeared to murder the influenza infection, per the CDC rules on the influenza infection. While utilizing harsher synthetic compounds like dye might be enticing, specialists propose holding off "until we know the impact on the texture's viability,. Discussing cleaning, you should load up on these family unit items that can execute coronavirus.

Are DIY Masks Effective?

Contingent upon the structure, masks can constrain the spread of a sickness from a tainted individual and shield the individual wearing them from disease.

On account of COVID-19, transmission of the infection is thought to happen basically through respiratory beads, which can land in others' mouths or noses when tainted individuals hack or wheeze. The beads can likewise pollute surfaces that others then touch before contacting their faces.

Here, essential careful masks — baggy, expendable masks — may be useful because if somebody who is debilitated is wearing one, their irresistible beads could be caught in the mask. Specialists and medical caretakers wearing such masks may likewise be secured fairly since they're probably going to be hacked or wheezed on.

However, specialists additionally presume the novel coronavirus, SARS-CoV-2, can wait noticeable all around in extremely little beads known as mist concentrates, which can be breathed in by individuals close by.

Rather than the N95 respirators, careful masks are not proposed to give security against vaporizers. careful masks "are intended to give boundary security against beads, anyway they are not controlled for particulate filtration productivity and they don't frame a satisfactory seal to the wearer's face to be depended upon for respiratory insurance."

Contrasted and careful masks or respirators, almost no exploration has been done on fabric masks.

Fabric face covers molded from family unit things or made at home from normal materials requiring little tod no effort can be utilized as an extra, willful general wellbeing measure.

What Materials Should You Use to Make a Mask?

- Cotton Fabric
- Shirt
- Handkerchief

Analysts at Cambridge University likewise contemplated which materials channel air best and can be utilized in an extemporized mask, finding that, beside careful masks, a pillowcase and a 100% cotton shirt were the most appropriate family unit materials.

To hold the mask to your face, you can utilize:

- Versatile
- Elastic groups
- String
- Fabric strips
- Fasteners

In what manner Should You Wear a Mask?

- fit cozily yet serenely against the side of the face
- be made sure about with ties or ear circles
- incorporate numerous layers of texture
- take into consideration breathing without limitation
- have the option to be washed and machine dried without harm or change to shape

What Are Some Things You Shouldn't Do?

Try not to put material face covers on little youngsters under the time of 2 or any individual who experiences difficulty breathing, is oblivious, debilitated or in any case unfit to take off the fabric face covering without help.

Don't to contact your eyes, nose, and mouth while taking off a fabric face covering and wash your hands following expelling.

Furthermore, don't utilize materials that are required for human services laborers. "The fabric face covers suggested are not careful masks or N-95 respirators," the office included. "Those are basic supplies that must keep on being held for social insurance laborers and other medical specialists on call."

Would it be a good idea for you to Wash Your Homemade Mask?

IT prompts routinely washing a hand crafted mask, yet how frequently you should wash them ought to be dictated by how regularly you are utilizing them. A clothes washer ought to appropriately disinfect a mask.

STEP BY STEP INSTRUCTIONS TO WEAR A MEDICAL FACE MASK

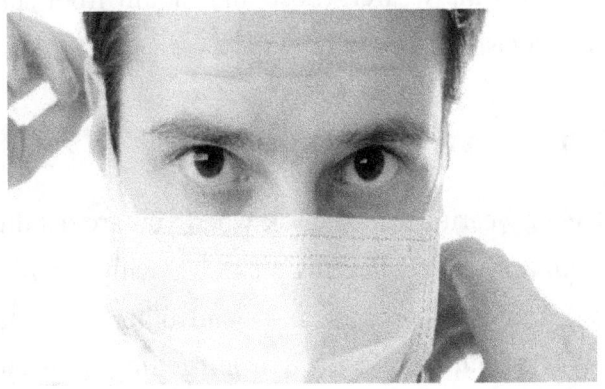

Face masks are one apparatus used for forestalling the spread of infection. They may likewise be called dental, confinement, laser, medical, technique, or careful masks. Face masks are baggy masks that spread the nose and mouth, and have ear circles or ties or groups at the rear of the head. There are a wide range of brands and they come in different hues. It is critical to utilize a face mask affirmed by the FDA.

What is a face mask utilized for

Facemasks help limit the spread of germs. At the point when somebody talks, hacks, or sniffles they may discharge little drops into the air that can taint others. If somebody is sick a face masks can lessen the quantity of germs that the wearer discharges and can shield others from getting wiped out. A face mask additionally shields the wearer's nose and mouth from sprinkles or splashes of body liquids.

When should a face mask be worn

Consider wearing a face mask when you are debilitated with a hack or wheezing sickness (with or without fever) and you hope to be around others. The face mask will help shield them from getting your sickness. Social insurance settings have specific principles for when individuals should wear face masks.

Step by step instructions to put on and evacuate a face mask

Dispensable face masks ought to be utilized once and afterward tossed in the rubbish. You ought to likewise evacuate and supplant masks when they become soggy.

Continuously adhere to item directions on use and capacity of the mask, and techniques for how to put on and evacuate a mask. If guidelines for putting on and evacuating the mask are not accessible, then follow the means underneath.

Step by step instructions to put on a face mask

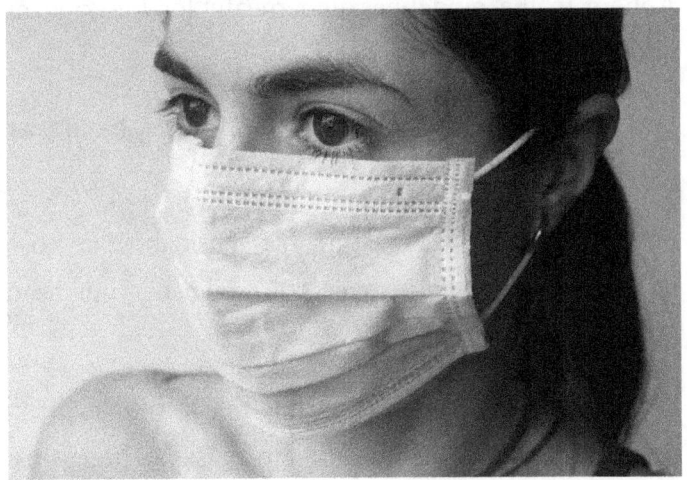

Clean your hands with cleanser and water or hand sanitizer before contacting the mask.

Expel a mask from the crate and ensure there are no undeniable tears or openings in either side of the mask.

Figure out which side of the mask is the top. The side of the mask that has a stiff bendable edge is the top and is intended to form to the state of your nose.

Figure out which side of the mask is the front. The hued side of the mask is normally the front and should face away from you, while the white side contacts your face.

Adhere to the guidelines underneath for the kind of mask you are utilizing.

Face Mask with Ear circles: Hold the mask by the ear circles. Spot a circle around every ear.

Face Mask with Ties: Bring the mask to your nose level and spot the ties over the crown of your head and secure with a bow.

Face Mask with Bands: Hold the mask in your grasp with the nosepiece or top of the mask at fingertips, permitting the headbands to hang uninhibitedly underneath hands. Carry the mask to your nose level and pull the top lash over your head with the goal that it rests over the crown of your head. Pull the base tie over your head so it rests at the scruff of your neck.

Form or squeeze the stiff edge to the state of your nose.

If utilizing a face mask with ties: Then take the base ties, one in each hand, and secure with a bow at the scruff of your neck.

Pull the base of the mask over your mouth and jaw.

Instructions to expel a face mask

Clean your hands with cleanser and water or hand sanitizer before contacting the mask. Avoid contacting the front of the mask. The front of the mask is debased. Just touch the ear circles/ties/band. Follow the directions underneath for the sort of mask you are utilizing.

Face Mask with Ear circles: Hold both of the ear circles and delicately lift and evacuate the mask.

Face Mask with Ties: Untie the base bow first then unfasten the top bow and pull the mask away from you as the ties are released.

Face Mask with Bands: Lift the base tie over your head first then force the top tie over your head.

Toss the mask in the rubbish. Clean your hands with cleanser and water or hand sanitizer.

There's a decent possibility you've never needed to stress over appropriately covering your nose and mouth before now — except if you've been a patient in a clinic, or work in medication or development. Notwithstanding, careful face masks just as face material face covers bought on the web or made at home are turning into a need during the novel coronavirus pandemic that has influenced Americans in every one of the 50 states.

Authorities at the Centers for Disease Control and Prevention are right now suggesting that everybody wear face covers out in the open — and pioneers in networks and states may likewise be ordering that you do as such. As of late, New York Governor Andrew Cuomo passed new council requesting that occupants wear a face mask when social removing measures aren't conceivable, remembering for open vehicle and inside fundamental organizations. Before long, pioneers in Southern California passed comparative direction with more grounded proposals for basic specialists on the clock, as did authorities in Pennsylvania.

Be that as it may, since a large portion of us are new to wearing face masks, we don't generally have the foggiest idea how to wear and deal with them effectively. So Good Housekeeping collected a board of irresistible sickness pros and scholastic specialists to walk you through how to appropriately wear a face mask. These specialists from driving establishments and emergency clinics in three different states are sharing their tips for keeping your face mask as sterile as could be expected under the circumstances, just as directions for how you put them on and take them off without presenting yourself to viral microscopic organisms. Here's the manner by which to evade normal wellbeing slips up when wearing a face mask.

The correct method to wear a medical or natively constructed mask:

Rodney Rohde, Ph.D., the partner senior member for look into for the College of Health Professions at Texas State University, says you ought to consistently wash your hands before taking care of any mask (this likewise applies to face covers, as well!). Taking care of within your mask with unwashed hands, regardless of whether you've bought it or you've sewn it yourself, adds to the hazard that you could take in microscopic organisms upon first use, successfully counterbalancing any sort of security it might offer you in any case.

Gonzalo Bearman, M.D., an emergency clinic disease transmission specialist at VCU Health and the seat of the Division of Infectious Diseases at Virginia Commonwealth University, says this is the right bit by bit process for wearing a medical mask or custom made fabric mask.

Get your mask by its ear circles. Without contacting the mask itself, bring the circles up to your ears, making sure about them as firmly as could be expected under the circumstances. If the mask is outfitted with ties rather than circles, tie the upper pair around the back crown of your head, then the second pair around the scruff of your neck.

Be certain that it covers your nose and your mouth. The mask shields you from regurgitating any microscopic organisms into the air by covering your nose and your mouth, Dr. Bearman clarifies. Dr. Rohde says wearing a medical mask appropriately may likewise give slight insurance if you want to get an opportunity at shielding yourself from any close by particles in your region.

Alter the attack of the mask to guarantee your jawline is secured. You can pull the mask around the base of your jawline, if conceivable. Tucking your mask underneath the jawline is a surefire approach to forestall the danger of changing it when you go out, Dr. Bearman includes.

Secure the mask around the extension of your nose. A few masks come outfitted with a metal tab exactly where the scaffold ought to be (if you feel a metal tab on your jaw, you'll realize your mask is topsy turvy).

Make certain to squeeze this into place with the goal that the highest point of the mask feels cozy to your face. Regardless of whether there is no metal tab, attempt your best to guarantee it won't descend your nose later.

Try to modify where required. Careful masks can't sift through all microscopic organisms, dissimilar to N95 masks utilized by social insurance experts, so you shouldn't stress a lot over holes between your face and the mask. "You simply need to ensure it best accommodates your face and has minimal measure of holes for air to channel through as could be expected under the circumstances," Dr. Bearman clarifies.

Robert Amler, M.D., the senior member of the school of wellbeing sciences and practices at New York Medical College, says there's another method to guarantee your face mask is cozy. "Regardless of whether it's a careful mask or fabric covering, when you put it on and secure it, wind your head to and fro, sideways, here and there to check whether the fit stays cozy every which way," he shares.

When removing the mask, you'll need to make certain to deal with it just by indistinguishable circles or ties from you did when you put it on. "Do whatever it takes not to contact the front or within the face mask when you're taking it off or when you're wearing it, as this can taint your hand with any microscopic organisms you've selected up while out in the open," Dr. Bearman clarifies.

Which side of a careful mask is the outside?

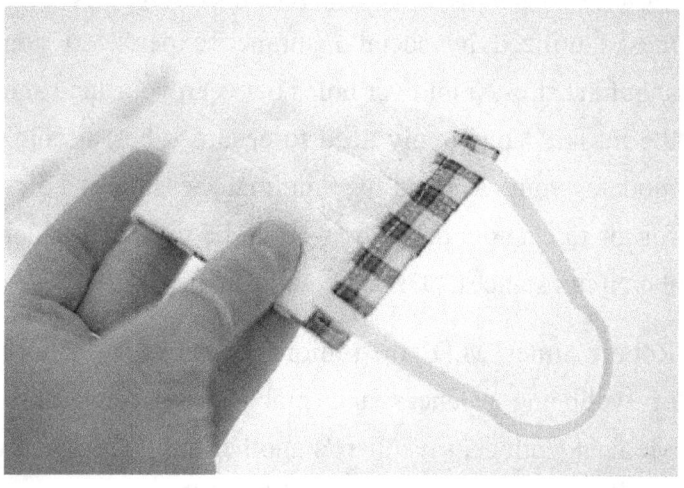

If you have bought a medical-grade careful mask, you might be pondering which side of the mask should be outwardly. While only one out of every odd producer follows a similar style, Dr. Rohde says that generally the side of the mask that is shaded is the outside of the mask. "If you look at the mask intently, you may have the option to see one side of the mask may really say 'inside' or 'outer' which causes you comprehend which part conflicts with your face," he clarifies. "For the greater part of the careful masks I've worn working in general wellbeing, the shading is confronting outwards."

Instructions to wear a DIY face covering:

If you don't approach a careful mask or a hand-sewn mask, a material face covering will in any case have the option to keep you from spreading microscopic organisms by means of respiratory beads out in the open spaces. "Utilizing a handkerchief is most likely better than nothing if you don't have a legitimate careful mask or a sewn face mask," Dr. Bearman says. "None of the masks are medical evaluation, and any holes are less significant, as these are intended to forestall beads and not mist concentrates. COVID-19 has been appeared to transmit with greater particles in beads and not by means of mist concentrates in ordinary spaces outside of emergency clinics." Plus, a face covering may go about as a human "hound cone" in that it reminds you to abstain from contacting your face.

Dr. Amler says you should fit a fabric covering similarly as you would deal with a mask. "Fabric covers, as careful masks, ought to be fitted cozily around your nose and mouth," he clarifies. "Once more, similar to a careful mask, a fabric covering should be made sure about in the rear of your head so it sits cozily against your face."

In what capacity would it be a good idea for me to clean my face mask?

After you've securely expelled your mask or covers by taking care of its ties or circles, Dr. Bearman says you ought to discard any careful masks, as these are made for single utilize as it were. You shouldn't endeavor to clean careful masks at home; some human services suppliers might be doing as such because of supply deficiencies, however all specialists don't suggest you do as such at home.

There isn't any solid information on how you should wash material covers, yet Carolyn Forte, Director of the Good Housekeeping Institute Cleaning Lab, proposes that all face masks ought to be washed with boiling water in the clothes washer, and tumble dried on high warmth.

If you have to store your fabric covering at home before washing it, put it in a dry paper pack if conceivable. Dr. Bearman clarifies that the dampness inside the face masks need to dry out, and it may not do as such in a shut box. Dr. Rohde adds that it's ideal to have a few material masks that you can cycle between so as to abstain from washing your fabric mask every single time you head outside.

STEPS AND STEPS INSTRUCTION ON HOW TO MAKE MEDICAL FACE MASK

———— ♦ ◇ ♦ ————

Not certain how to wear or clean the masks? We answer those inquiries under the mask-production guidelines.

Materials you'll require

- 2 bits of tight-weave cotton texture, 9 x 6 inches (per mask)
- 4 portions of texture, 2 x 16 inches (per mask)
- Ruler
- Sewing machine OR needle and string
- Pencil or marker
- Scissors
- A bunch of sewing pins
- Iron

Make your mask

1. Cut your texture into two 9 x 6-inch square shapes. Spot them on one another.
2. On the highest point of the 9-inch side, pin or imprint a 2-inch opening in the focal point of the top edge of the 9-inch side, between the 3.5-and 5.5-inch focuses, along the top edge. Then, sew the edges on either side of where you stuck or denoted the opening. You'll require that 2-inch opening to turn the mask right side out.
3. Sew the other three sides of the mask shut, as well.
4. Turn the mask right side out through the 2-inch opening you left on the top. Then, press the mask with an iron to dispose of wrinkles.
5. Line your ruler up vertically along the 6-inch side of the mask. Beginning at the 1.5-inch line, pin where you'll sew your creases down the side. These creases help the mask stretch.

Pin again at the 2-, 3-, 3.5-, 4.5-and 5-inch lines.

6. Bring the pin at the 1.5-inch line down to the 2-inch line, and presto, you've made a crease! Rehash with the 3-inch to the 3.5-inch and the

4.5-inch to the 5-inch line. Pin your new creases, and rehash on the opposite side.
7. Close the sides of your mask up so the creases are laid level.

Make mask ties

1. Cut four portions of texture, 2 inches wide by 16 inches in length.
2. Overlap them fifty-fifty the long way.
3. Turn them under 1/4-inch on the long side.
4. Iron them set up, then join the long side shut.
5. Pin each bind to a side of the mask.
6. Sew around the edge of the mask again so the ties are connected - and now you've finished your mask.

If you don't have the foggiest idea how to sew

Mask FAQs

How would I wear it?

Masks are just successful if you wear them appropriately. The World Health Organization has the how-to:

- Wash your hands for 20 seconds with cleanser and water before contacting or putting on the mask.
- Ensure your whole nose and mouth are secured when you put it on.
- Abstain from contacting the mask while you're out - this can defile it.
- Try not to take the mask off while you're openly.
- To take it off once you return, loosen it from the back - don't contact its front.
- You ought to promptly wash the mask subsequent to returning so it doesn't pollute your things.
- Wash your hands following you've taken it off, and again after you've washed the mask.

Are masks even powerful?

Natively constructed mask contemplates have indicated that they're significantly less powerful than careful masks - and they're positively no swap for the basic N95 respirators medicinal services laborers must wear to treat patients.

They offer a physical obstruction from viral particles, he stated, however they don't have the channels that N95 respirators do.

However, they're superior to nothing, particularly for individuals who just go out in broad daylight to make a snappy excursion to the market or drug store, said Anna Davies and Raina MacIntyre, general wellbeing specialists and creators of two separate examinations on the viability of fabric mask.

It's essential to note, however, that masks can't supplant social removing measures. Keeping up at any rate six feet of good ways from others and remaining at home however much as could be expected is as yet the most ideal approach to forestall the spread of the infection.

How would you clean them?

You ought to wash the masks when each utilization to clear off any germs you may have gotten in broad daylight. Hand wash the masks or put them in a work wash sack in the clothes washer so they don't self-destruct, and utilize a high warmth setting.

Imagine a scenario in which my specialty store is shut or out of provisions.

Crafters on Etsy aren't sold out of face masks yet. It's difficult to observe how compelling these masks are since you didn't create them yourself, however you can contrast them with our mask instructional exercise before you purchase - does it spread your nose and mouth? Are there creases? Will it firmly seal around your face?

You likely don't have to purchase in excess of a couple of masks - doctors suggest that just a single individual from every family unit gets things done out in the open.

It might take longer than expected to transport the masks, so know about this when you purchase.

Furthermore, make certain to wash the masks before you wear them.

If you can't get to masks by any means, then continue washing your hands, keeping up good ways from others and following other social separating measures. Remaining at home is the best resistance against coronavirus, all things considered.

TYPES OF MEDICAL FACE MASK

What are the three essential kinds of face masks?

At the point when you catch wind of face masks for COVID-19 counteraction, it's commonly three sorts:

- homemade fabric face mask
- surgical mask
- N95 respirator

How about we investigate every one of them in somewhat more detail underneath.

Homemade Fabric Face Masks

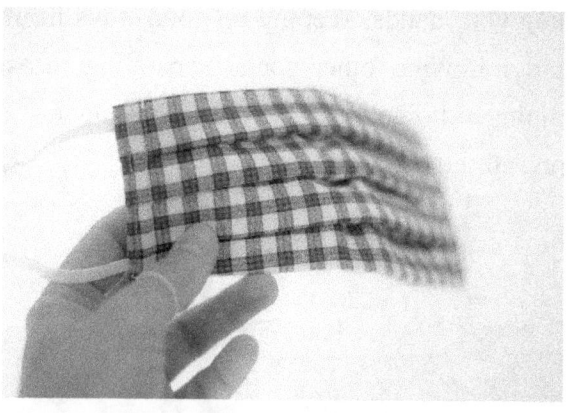

To keep the spread of the infection from individuals without manifestations, the Centers for Disease Control and Prevention (CDC) is presently recommending Trusted Source that everybody wears material face masks, for example, natively constructed face masks Trusted Source, while in broad daylight places where it's difficult to keep up a 6-foot good ways from others. This suggestion is notwithstanding proceeded with social separating and appropriate cleanliness rehearses.

Proposals include:

Wear material face masks in open settings, particularly in territories of significant network based transmission, for example, supermarkets and drug stores.

Try not to put material face masks on youngsters younger than 2, individuals who experience difficulty breathing, individuals who are oblivious, or individuals who can't evacuate the mask all alone.

Use fabric face masks as opposed to careful masks or N95 respirators, as these basic supplies must be saved for medicinal services laborers and other medical specialists on call.

Medicinal services experts should practice extraordinary alert when utilizing custom made face masks.

These masks ought to ideally be utilized in blend with a face shield that covers the whole front and sides of the face and stretches out to the jaw or underneath.

NOTE: Wash custom made fabric masks after each utilization. While evacuating, be mindful so as not to contact your eyes, nose, and mouth. Wash hands following expelling.

Advantages of homemade face masks

Fabric face masks can be made at home from normal materials, so there's a boundless stockpile.

They may bring down the danger of individuals without side effects transmitting the infection through talking, hacking, or wheezing.

They're better than not utilizing any mask and offer some security, particularly where social separating is difficult to keep up.

Dangers of homemade face masks

They may give a misguided feeling that all is well and good. While hand crafted face masks offer some level of security, they offer significantly less assurance than careful masks or respirators. One 2008 study Trusted

Source showed that hand crafted face masks might be half as powerful as careful masks and up to multiple times less successful than N95 respirators.

They don't swap or lessen the requirement for other defensive measures. Legitimate cleanliness practices and social separating are as yet the best techniques for protecting yourself.

Surgical masks

Surgical masks are dispensable, baggy face masks that spread your nose, mouth, and jaw. They're normally used to:

- Shield the wearer from showers, sprinkles, and enormous molecule beads
- Forestall the spread of conceivably irresistible respiratory emissions from the wearer to other people
- Surgical masks can fluctuate in structure, however the mask itself is frequently level and rectangular fit as a fiddle with creases or overlays. The highest point of the mask contains a metal strip that can be framed to your nose.
- Versatile groups or long, straight ties help hold a careful mask set up while you're wearing it.

These can either be circled behind your ears or tied behind your head.

N95 respirators

A N95 respirator is an all the more tight-fitting face mask. Notwithstanding sprinkles, splashes, and huge beads, this respirator can likewise sift through 95 percent Trusted Source of exceptionally little particles. This incorporates infections and microbes.

The respirator itself is commonly round or oval fit as a fiddle and is intended to frame a tight seal to your face. Versatile groups help hold it solidly to your face. A few sorts may have a connection called an exhalation valve, which can help with breathing and the development of warmth and dampness.

N95 respirators aren't one-size-fits-all. They really should be fit-tried before use to ensure that a legitimate seal is shaped. If the mask doesn't seal viably to your face, you won't get the suitable assurance.

In the wake of being fit-tried, clients of N95 respirators must keep on playing out a seal check each time they put one on. It's additionally imperative to take note of that a tight seal can't be accomplished in certain gatherings. These incorporate kids and individuals with facial hair.

BENEFIT OF MEDICAL FACE MASK

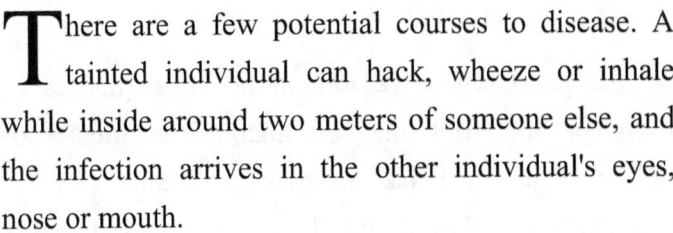

There are a few potential courses to disease. A tainted individual can hack, wheeze or inhale while inside around two meters of someone else, and the infection arrives in the other individual's eyes, nose or mouth.

Another course is the point at which a contaminated individual hacks or wheezes onto their hand or onto a surface. The uninfected individual then shakes the hand or contacts the surface, and moves the infection to their own eye, nose or mouth.

It is conceivable that a contaminated individual can likewise hack or wheeze to make an airborne spread past the nearby contact run – however it is questionable whether this last course is a significant methods for transmission.

We don't have the foggiest idea how much transmission happens by every one of these courses for COVID-19. It's additionally muddled how much insurance a mask would offer for each situation.

Current best proof

To determine this inquiry, we dissected 14 randomized preliminaries of mask wearing and disease for flu like ailments. (There are no randomized preliminaries including COVID-19 itself, so all the better we can do is take a gander at comparable ailments.)

At the point when we joined the consequences of these preliminaries that considered the impact of masks versus no masks in social insurance laborers and everyone, they didn't show that wearing masks prompts any significant decrease of flu like ailment. Be that as it may, the examinations were too little to even think about ruling out a minor impact for masks.

For what reason don't masks secure the wearer?

There are a few potential reasons why masks don't offer significant security. To begin with, masks may not do much without eye insurance. We know from creature and research center examinations that flu or different coronaviruses can enter the eyes and travel to the nose and into the respiratory framework.

While standard and extraordinary masks give inadequate insurance, exceptional masks joined with goggles seem to give total assurance in research center investigations. Be that as it may, there are no investigations in genuine circumstances estimating the after-effects of consolidated mask and eyewear.

The clear insignificant effect of wearing masks may likewise be because individuals didn't utilize them appropriately. For instance, one investigation discovered not exactly 50% of the members wore them "more often than not". Individuals may likewise wear masks improperly, or contact a debased piece of the mask while evacuating it and move the infection to their hand, then their eyes and therefore to the nose.

Masks may likewise give a misguided sensation that all is well and good, which means wearers may do more hazardous things, for example, going into swarmed spaces and places.

Do masks secure others?

Could masks shield others from the infection that may have been spread by the mask wearer? An ongoing Hong Kong research facility study discovered some proof masks may forestall the spread of infections from the wearer.

They took individuals with flu like side effects, gave half of them masks and a large portion of no masks, and for 30 minutes gathered infections from the air they inhaled out, including hacks.

Masks reduced the measures of beads and pressurized canned products containing perceivable measures of infection. Be that as it may, just 17 of the 111 subjects had a coronavirus, and these were not the SARS-CoV-2 coronavirus. While the investigation is promising, it should be rehashed desperately.

We likewise don't have the foggiest idea how this decrease of vaporizers and beads means decrease of contaminations in reality. If there is an impact, it might be weakened by a few factors, for example, sick individuals who don't wear a mask and "well" individuals who have no manifestations yet are as yet conveying and spreading the infection.

Masks for a few?

If wearing masks does considerably decrease the spread of the disease to other people, what would it be advisable for us to do? We could ask everybody with any respiratory side effects to wear masks out in the open. That could enhance different systems, for example, social separating, testing, following and following to lessen transmission.

To likewise catch contaminated individuals without manifestations, we could request that everybody wear masks in indoor open spaces. Outside is increasingly difficult, since the vast majority present next to zero hazard. Maybe, as we lessen limitations, masks could likewise be required at some open air swarm occasions, for example, games or shows.

Another chance is a "2 x 2" rule: if you are outside and inside 2 meters of others for over 2 minutes you have to wear a mask.

Mask wearing for the potentially tainted, to forestall spreading the disease, warrants thorough and fast examination. It could be another option or an enhancement to social separating, hand cleanliness, testing, and lockdowns.

DIY MEDICAL FACE MASK PATTERN

——————— ◆◇◆ ———————

Since the episode of the ongoing pandemic infection, I have been culminating and extemporizing this face mask example to incorporate all the highlights that expected to battle against the spread of the illness. One of the highlights incorporates including an opening or pocket for channel media to make the face mask increasingly compelling. Besides, a nose clip (otherwise known as nose wire) is included at the top edge of the face mask to give a superior seal at the nose connect region. Thirdly, because of deficiencies of versatile band and furthermore because of the solace of the wearability, head tie made out of shoelace and shirt yarn are prescribed to use here. Fourthly, a sewing video is made for a superior perspective on the sewing procedure.

You may peruse the accompanying dated updates for the subtleties that have been made to this example, some enormous and some little changes to consummate the example. I am happy to get messages and remarks from all channels, they are disclosing to me that numerous clinics and nearby specialists have requested that their kin sew from the Craft Passion face mask design because this custom made face mask gives incredible inclusion and seal. I trust my little modest exertion and the hand crafted face mask design makes a gigantic difference to the world. Ultimately, not neglecting to thank you for sewing face masks and give to the individuals who required it, you are all gift from heaven blessed messengers.

With exceptionally infectious coronavirus (COVID19) quickly spreading all through the world, numerous individuals are looking for careful masks to ensure against this risky sickness.

The abrupt increment sought after for "Individual Protective Equipment" (PPE) and the interfered with supply lines in China have prompted a basic lack of little molecule sifting face masks (N-95s) and fitted rectangular wheeze monitors ("careful masks").

News reports, fittingly trying to save constrained supplies of these dispensable things for medical foundations, have been asking individuals not to buy these things. Open authorities have been cited recommending that face covers can't help forestall the spread of this new infection.

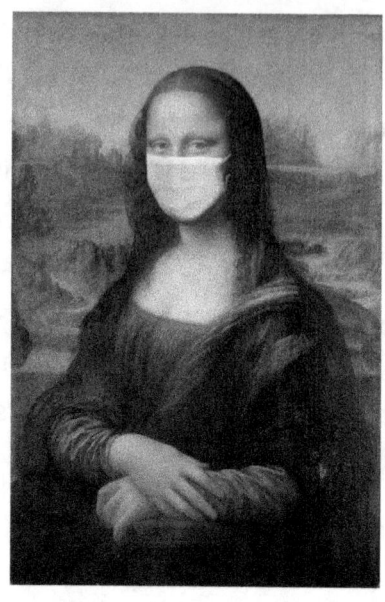

In all actuality increasingly confounded:

COVID19 is spread from individual to-individual in beads of dampness, bodily fluid and spit from individuals with contaminations. Hacking, wheezing, and even ordinary breathing put these infection particles into the air. One sniffle can put out a large number of beads.

Individuals standing under 6 feet away may get secured with these infection particles while they are still noticeable all around. After the beads fall, the infection particles can stay dynamic for as long as nine days.

Contamination happens when somebody takes in airborne beads, or when they contact their mouth, nose or eyes with hands canvassed in infection particles that have dropped out of the air onto counters, hand rails, floors or different surfaces.

Wearing a face mask assists prevent with peopling from getting contaminated in two different ways:

- By blocking most airborne beads loaded up with infection from being breathed in
- By preventing the wearer from contacting their own mouths and noses.

Studies have demonstrated that medical expert utilizing careful face masks effectively get 80% less contaminations than the individuals who don't.

So why the blended messages?

In the first place, because the insurance possibly comes when the masks are utilized appropriately. They should be put on spotless, taken off cautiously, and matched with thorough hand washing, and the control not to contact the face.

Second, because holes around the masks and between the strands in the masks, even in business careful masks, are too huge to even consider blocking all infections. Wheeze and hack beads are typically somewhere in the range of 7 and 100 microns. Careful masks and some fabric masks will square 7 micron particles yet the COVID19 infection particles are 0.06 to 0.14 microns.

So for what reason would it be a good idea for you to make your own face masks?

1) In the occasion you become wiped out, having an inventory of masks at home will give some degree of insurance to loved ones while you look for medical counsel. It will absolutely be superior to no mask by any stretch of the imagination (see look into notes).
2) By making your own, and ideally for loved ones, you will be diminishing interest on constrained supplies of modernly made, disposables, which are urgently required by emergency clinics and nursing homes.
3) These agreeable, bended molded masks rest nearer to the face, with less holes, than rectangular careful masks.
4) Our custom made plans are launderable, making them naturally benevolent.

Supplies:

Mask 1 is fitted, with 2 layers of texture and a pocket between them for a discretionary channel (see look into joins for information on channels). It is hung on by versatile ear circles. Flexible can likewise be strung to fit around the head.

Mask 2 is fitted, with 2 layers yet no pocket, and is simpler to make.

Crease stipends are ¼" except if noted

MASK 1 and 2 supplies (kid, standard and huge size):

- 8" x 12" texture external layer
- 8" x 12" texture lining layer
- 3" bit of delicate wire (this can be enlivening wire as appeared, picture wire, or a funnel cleaner multiplied over)
- approx. 22" of flexible string (youngster size length 10", ordinary size length 11-12", huge size length 13")

WHAT KIND OF FABRIC?

You can pick any firmly woven cotton or cotton/poly texture you like. Hold it up to the light to perceive how tight the weave is. Utilize a similar texture for external and coating if you need, or utilize different ones to assist you with recollecting which side is perfect and which messy.

The examination (see joins toward the end) shows 100% cotton having some viability. Cotton/polyester mixes may have extra properties of repulsing water, improving them hindrances to shield beads from splashing through external layers.

Try not to utilize stretchy, sequined or velvet material.

Wash all textures before sewing to pre-shrivel, and to guarantee you are working with the most sterile materials conceivable.

Stage 1: Pattern, Cut, Center Seam

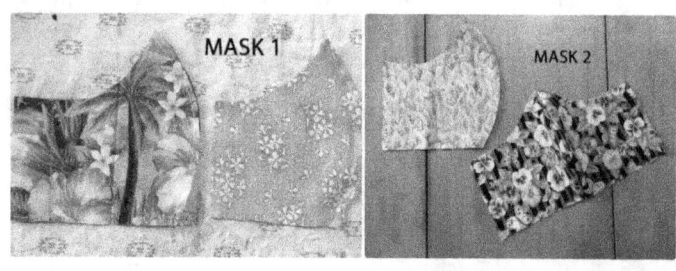

Print out PDF paper pattern piece(s) at genuine size on 8.5" x 11" paper. For MASK 1 print record called "Mask 1 reg size pattern". It has 2 pieces: An (external) and B (lining) . For MASK 2, print either "Mask 2 reg size pattern" or "Mask 2 enormous pattern" or "Mask 2 kid pattern". It simply has one piece. Right now I don't have an enormous or kid size pattern for a Mask 1. Will deal with that. Cut out the paper pattern pieces.

ABOUT PRINTING THE PATTERNS:

- For those without a printer - open up the gridded pattern PDF so you can draw it yourself
- Ensure you print with the scene direction, not picture or it will come out excessively little.
- Here are the estimations for reference Don't worry around 1/8" minor departure from your printed patterns. There is squirm room in the plan:
    - ➢ Mask 1 piece An is 6 3/8" h x 5.25" w. at the base B is 6 3/8" h x 4.25" w at the base
    - ➢ Mask 2 kid is 5.25" h x 4 7/8" w and the base
    - ➢ Mask 2 ordinary is 6.25" h x 5.5" w at the base
    - ➢ Mask 2 huge is 6.75" h x 6" w at the base
- Instructables people group part Winko made versatile records for masks 1 and 2. Go to this

connection and open the pattern you need in your program. There is a drop down menu with print estimating alternatives, including an adaptable one.
- European paper size: I've been informed that the paper size in Europe is DIN4 and you have to alter the scale to 107%.

MASK 1

- Layer your textures right sides together.
- Pin pattern(s) to collapsed textures and cut two An and two B. Move the 2 dabs from pattern onto the two A pieces on wrong side of texture. Pencil a line between them gently on each piece.

MASK 2

- Layer your textures right sides together.
- Pin pattern piece to collapsed textures (external and covering). Cut 4.
- Sew focus bends of external layers, right sides together. Sew focus bends of covering layers, right sides together. Clasp the bended crease at

about ½" interims however not down to the crease.

Stage 2: MASK 1 Sides, Sleeves for Elastic

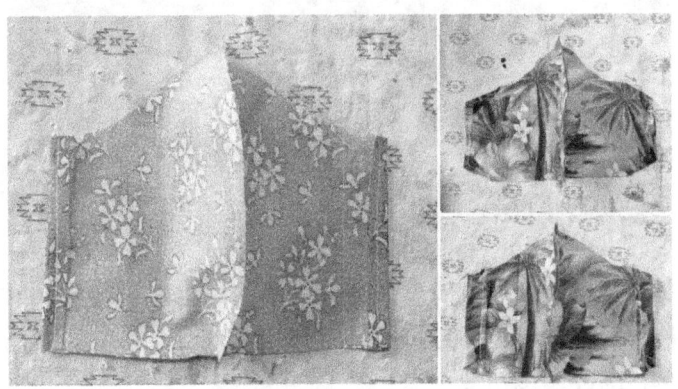

For MASK 1 (with pocket)

Crease straight sides of coating texture toward wrong side, and sew overlay down with straight line.

On external layer sides, crease top and base corners down, utilizing the specked lines on pattern and the moved spots as aides. Pin. Crease crude edge over and pin. Pressing helps keep this set up. Line along all the 3 overlap on each side, 1/8" from crease.

Make the sleeves for the flexible - With wrong side up, overlay calculated, sewed parts of the bargains up to the pencil line. Join down.

Stage 3: MASK 1 Connect Layers, Elastic

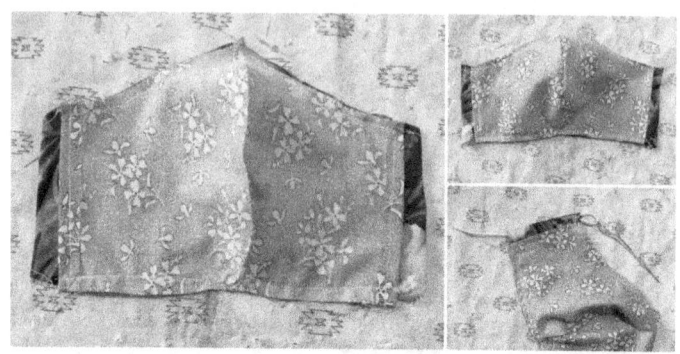

Lay internal layer over external layer, right sides looking in. Sew the top edge and the base edge. Clasp bended crease.

Turn right side out. Top line the top and base creases, 1/8" from edge. This will guarantee the two layers remain set up during washing.

Feed flexible through the sleeves (approx. 11" per side). A wire needle or little self locking pin can help feed it through.

Stage 4: MASK 1 Nose Wire, Elastic, Filter

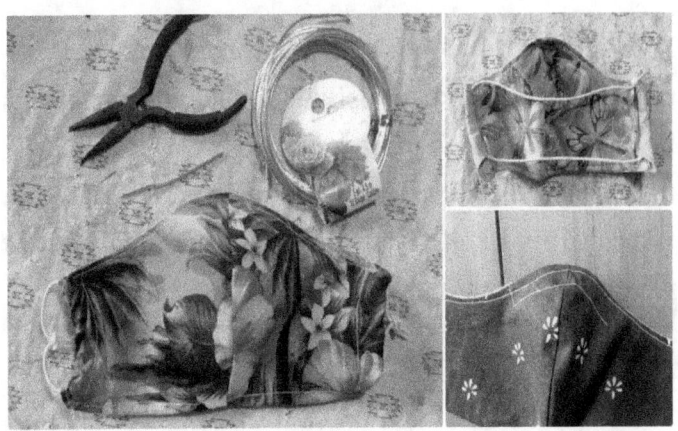

Make a channel to hold the nose wire by sewing a line 1/4" from the top line, reverberating the bend (2" on each side). Slide a 3"ish bit of wire into the space made (circle the closures first with pincers if they are sharp). Sew the parts of the bargains shut.

Tie parts of the bargains circles and fit mask to your head by tucking circles behind ears. Change hitches varying. It should fit cozily yet not pull on your ears. If wanted, you can cause the versatile to go around the rear of the head. Try not to slice the versatile down the middle. Feed each finish of the 16" length through the sleeves in a U shape. Tie together and fit mask. Alter tie varying for cozy fit.

Curve the wire to fit cozily over the extension of your nose.

Discretionary: If you have a reasonable channel material, you can build the sifting limit by slipping this material into the pocket between the external layer and the coating. Slice whatever channel material to fit varying. See look into notes for increasingly about what may be appropriate.

Stage 5: MASK 2 Instructions

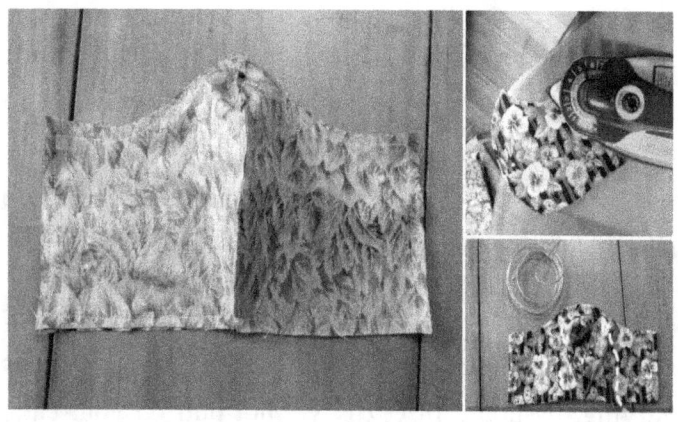

For MASK 2 (simpler, no pocket)

Pin right sides of external and covering layers confronting one another. Sew right around the edge, with the exception of a 1.5" hole on the base edge. Turn right side out and press.

Note - the pointy end of a pressing board is the ideal size and shape to press these masks on.

Sew the wire channel, 1/2" down from edge and 2" to each side of the inside crease. See picture.

Slide the wire through the turning opening, into the wire channel. Line the parts of the bargains shut so it won't move around when washed.

Top join 1/8" around the whole mask, shutting everything down turning opening as you do. Be cautious about the wire. You can avoid that area of top sewing if there isn't sufficient space to go over the wire.

Lay mask with arranging side on table and overlay 1" of each finish of the mask toward the middle. Stick and sew, making the versatile channels.

Individuals are getting inventive with regards to making natively constructed face masks and covers at home - from causing headbands with catches to forestall scraping around the ears to clear covers over the mouth so their lips can be perused. They're in any event, utilizing 3D printers to make face shields and mask frill. Face covers like these are currently a typical sight in markets, open transportation, drug stores and even in the city. A few states and provinces presently expect occupants to wear face masks out in the open with an end goal to slow the spread of the coronavirus.

We realize you should have questions, so we're separating what you have to think about creation, wearing, purchasing and giving masks, from hand-sewn masks to no-sew covers and even handkerchiefs appended to your ears with barrettes.

Custom made face masks will most likely be unable to shut out each molecule, and are not ensured to shield you from getting the coronavirus, yet they can help in certain conditions (more beneath). The extreme deficiency of N95 masks, which help ensure medical experts like specialists and attendants from gaining the coronavirus, has implied that normal residents required a choice to help moderate the spread. (Not long ago, the FDA affirmed a disinfection procedure for N95 masks to help adapt to the deficiency.)

Social separating on strolls and in stores, and that intensive hand-washing is as yet the most pushed medical guidance for sound individuals to abstain from procuring the coronavirus.

DIY MEDICAL FACE MASK FILTER

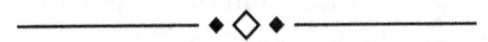

Stage 1: Gather the Supplies

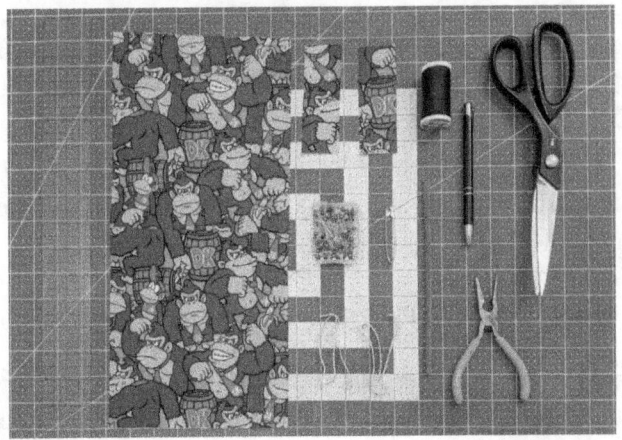

All that I Used:

Apparatuses:

- Sewing Machine
- Scissors
- Forceps
- Pins
- Iron

Supplies:

1 Piece of Cotton Fabric 15" x 7.5" - If your utilizing a printed texture with a directional print, ensure you cut this vertically like appeared in the image above to ensure your print doesn't wind up sideways. I really sorted mine out with 2 bits of texture to make one long piece since I was coming up short on texture so please overlook the extra crease :)

2 Bias Strips of Fabric 1.5" x 4"

1 Pipe Cleaner 7.5" long (you could likewise substitute with wire or skirt this progression if you don't need the mask to shape over your nose)

2 Strips of Elastic 9.75" long (If you can't discover flexible you could utilize long clasps, portions of texture or anything that would work to make sure about the mask over your ears)

String

Stage 2: Add a Zig Zag Stitch to the Short Sides

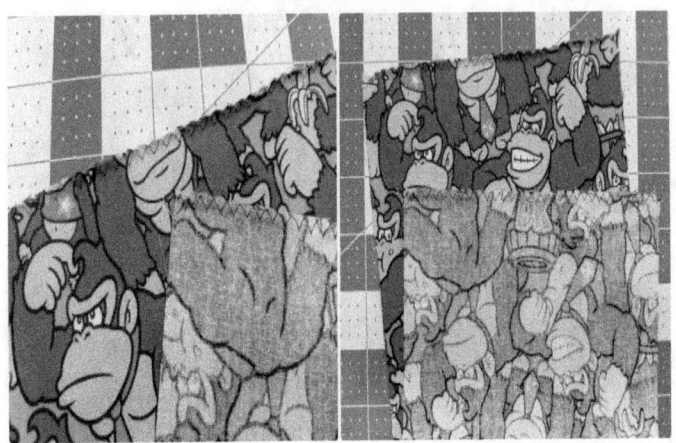

To secure sides of the texture, give them a perfect wrap up by including a crisscross line or if you have a serger, serge them. This solitary should be done to the 7.5" sides of the principle bit of texture.

Stage 3: Fold and Sew the Top of the Mask

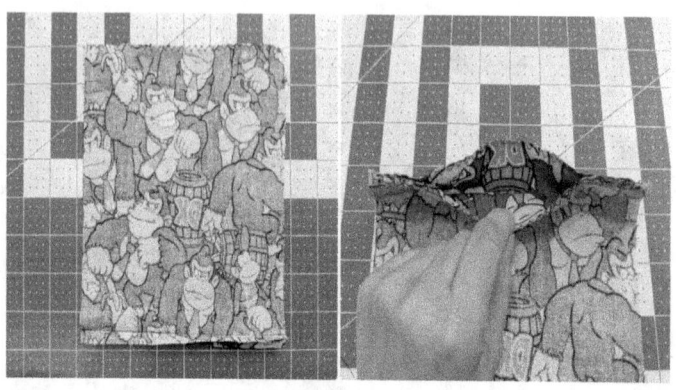

Overlap your fundamental bit of texture into equal parts with the correct sides together.

Pin the top crisscross edges together.

Sew 1/2" in on the two sides of the top crisscross edge with a 3/8" crease remittance, leaving a 4 1/2" hole in the middle. This hole will be the pocket opening for the channel.

Stage 4: Finish the Edge of the Pocket Opening

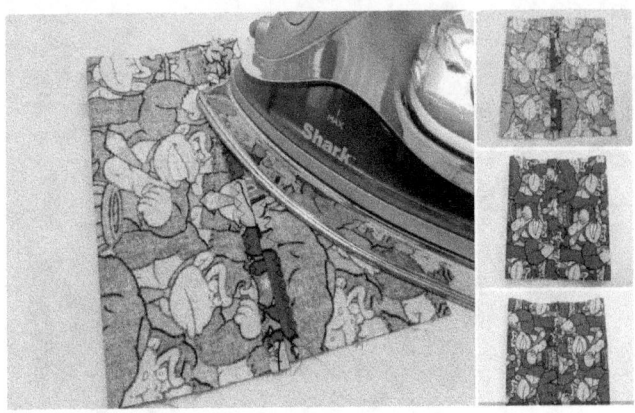

Focus the crease remittance and utilize an iron to press the crease stipend level.

Turn the mask right side out.

Add topstitching to the two sides of the crease. This ought to be around 1/8" from the crease and will hold the crease remittance level and set up.

Level your mask and position the crease/pocket opening 1/2" down from the top edge. To assist in the following stage you can squeeze this level and pin the open edges together.

Sew an edge line around the whole external edge as near the edge as could reasonably be expected, around 1/8".

Stage 5: Insert the Pipe Cleaner

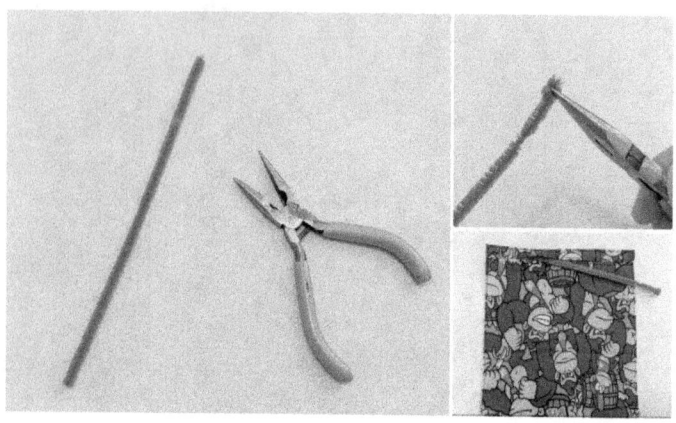

For these masks I utilized a funnel cleaner yet you could likewise utilize wire.

The wire should be 6 1/2" when embedded. I began with a 7 1/2" piece and utilized forceps to turn the edges a couple of times to balance them so they would not be pointy and jab a gap through the texture once wrapped up.

Addition the channel cleaner however the pocket opening and focus it at the top edge of the crease.

To secure it, sew directly over your past line on the top edge of the pocket opening crease. Your pocket should at present be open and useful.

Stage 6: Add the Pleats

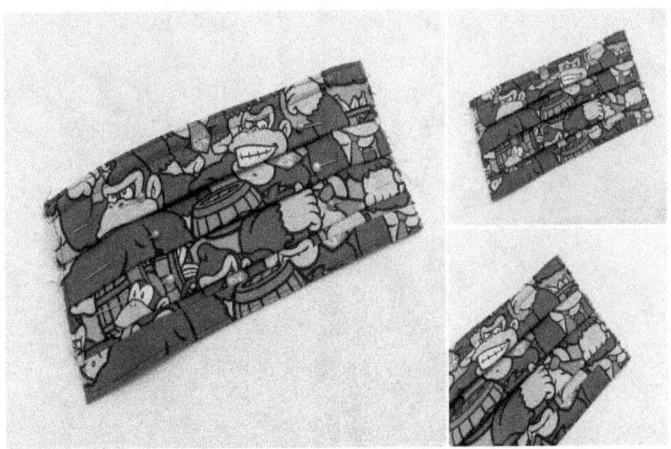

Working from the front of the mask (the back is the side with the pocket opening) include 3 creases. You could include anyway numerous you need however this is the manner by which I sewed mine.

I made my creases around 1/2" wide and when I was done my sides estimated 3 1/2"

Pin the creases set up and iron them level.

Sew along the whole side with a 1/8" edge fasten to keep the creases set up and rehash for the two sides.

Stage 7: Add the Bias Binding

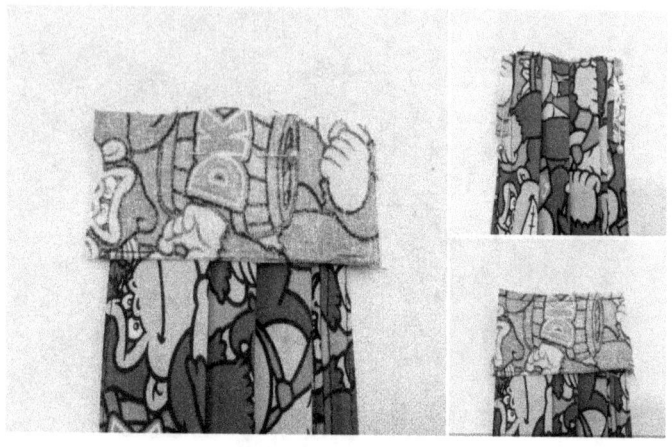

Focus one segment of inclination to the rear of one of the creased sides with the correct sides together, and pin set up. You ought to have 1/4" abundance on the two sides.

Crease the 1/4" abundance over to the front of the mask and pin set up.

Sew the inclination to the mask utilizing a 1/8" edge line.

Rehash these means for the contrary side.

Overlap the predisposition tape out and press the 1/4" overlays down with an iron.

Rehash for the two sides.

To complete the bound edges, overlap the predisposition in towards the mask multiple times and pin set up. You ought to have decent collapsed edges. This coupling will make a passage for your flexible to slide through.

Sew along the inward edge of the official with a 1/8" edge join so keep the authoritative set up and give you space for the versatile. Rehash for the two sides.

Stage 8: Add the Elastic

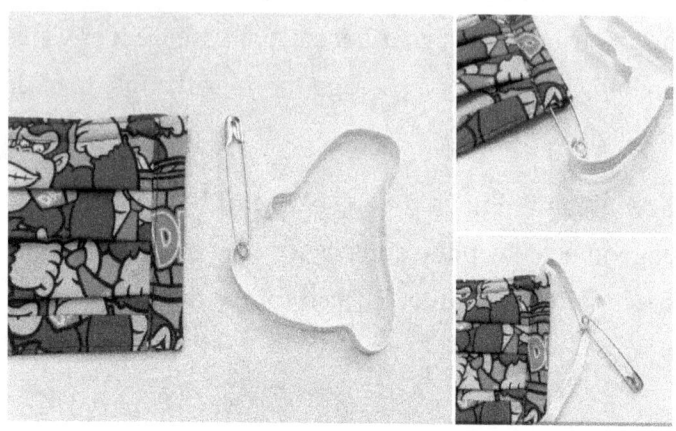

Take 1 flexible strip and join one end to a self locking pin.

Slide the self clasping pin through one side of the official and push it completely through.

To make sure about your versatile, twofold bunch the closures so they are tight.

To complete, maneuver your flexible to slide the bunch into the official. This will hide the flexible bunch. This part can be somewhat dubious relying upon the size of flexible you are utilizing.

Rehash for the contrary side.

Stage 9: Wear and Enjoy!

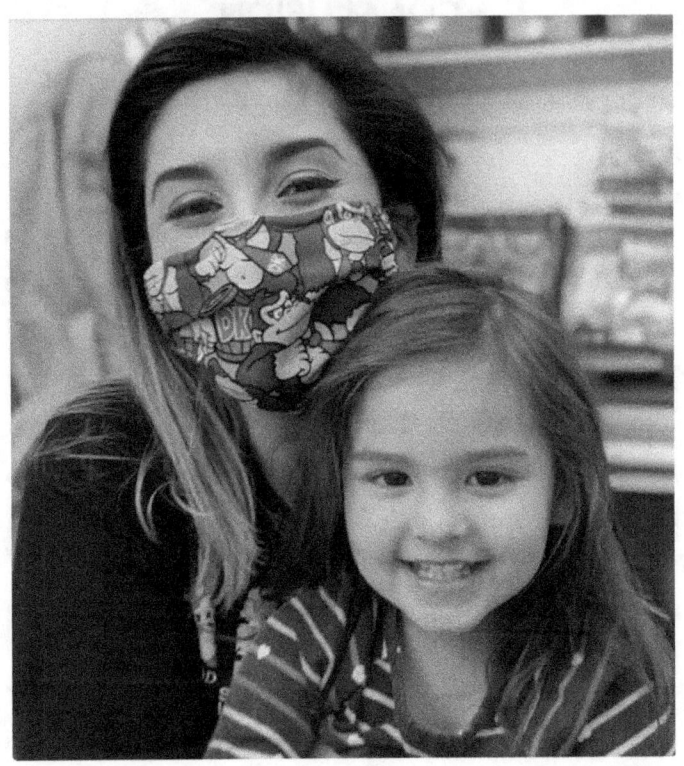

Wear and Enjoy!

What's more, that is it! Presently you can wear your new mask and appreciate it! Make some for your loved ones or give them to any individual who needs them!

CONCLUSION

———— ◆◇◆ ————

An extraordinary method to spoil yourself is to treat your face with fixings that will breath life into it back. Masks are an overall quite fast method for accomplishing and keeping up great skin. You can likewise make DIY masks at home with fixings at home. They are less expensive, simpler and easy to make. Here are a couple DIY face masks that you can pursue different skin issues:

1. Hydrating Honey Mask

If your skin has been feeling dry and dull from workaholic behavior or cruel climate all you need is something that will saturate your skin.

Fixings You Need:

- Nectar
- Rosewater
- Avocado

Blend these fixings well and leave it on your face for 15-30 minutes. Let the fixings drench into your skin well. Wash it off and you will see discernibly smooth and splendid skin.

2. Battle That Acne

Skin inflammation can result from contamination that can obstruct your pores, along these lines, setting off your skin to breakout. Try not to stress because you can without much of a stretch get them dry inside days.

Fixings You Need:

- Yogurt
- Turmeric
- Lemon

This is one of the most established DIY insider facts in history for clear skin. If you have skin break out inclined or slick skin, this face pack will deal with it. Yogurt has hostile to bacterial properties though turmeric dries out skin inflammation in this manner dispensing with them. Then again, lemon will help any past skin break out scars and make your skin look splendid and reasonable.

3. Fix Those Pores

Pores can be a genuine wellspring of trouble. They are difficult to stow away even with cosmetics on because your make will begin to look flaky sooner or later if you have large pores on your skin. You can attempt a DIY Mask to fix them and reestablish infant delicate skin.

Fixings You Need

- Egg White
- Lemon

Blend these fixings well and leave them on your face until they dry. Then you can either wash it off or strip it off contingent upon the consistency of the mask. Egg white will fix pores just as expel contaminations and pimples that will give you a normally impeccable shine up!

4. Blocked Skin

Blocked skin can bring about skin inflammation breakouts reliably. It tends to be caused because of an unfortunate eating routine, ill-advised resting pattern or warm climate. Be that as it may, there is a face mask for everything when you DIY it.

Fixings You Need

- Rose Water
- Aloe Vera
- Cucumber

Blend these fixings and subsequent to washing your face with your standard chemical put the blend on your face. Leave it on your face for 15-20 minutes. Wash it off. Do this each other day if your skin is exceptionally risky else you can do this each once in seven days. It will permit your skin to chill off and discharge poisons that are causing clog.

5. Light up It Up

Dull skin can be brought about by restlessness, exhausting and not take adequate consideration of your skin. You can light up and evacuate dead cells with assistance of the most fundamental fixings in your kitchen.

Fixings You Need

- Earthy colored Sugar
- Nectar
- Virgin Olive Oil

Blend these fixings in sums that you have scour like consistency. Apply it on your face and delicately rub it everywhere. Wash off the face a while later to uncover the enchantment of this straightforward hydrating mask. Additional advantage: You can likewise utilize it all the rage.

6. Switch Aging

If you have almost negligible differences or wrinkles on your face it is because of the absence of hydration and dampness. Notwithstanding, there are specific fixings that will assist you with hindering the procedure and evacuate scarcely discernible differences.

Fixings You Need

- Cocoa Powder
- Cream
- Nectar

Blend these fixings and leave the blend on your face for 20-30 minutes. By applying this face mask on your face every now and again you will see a colossal difference in your appearance. This face mask is pressed with enemies of oxidants and is known for collagen boosting system.

For each skin issue, there is a mask. You can likewise mess with different fixings all alone to suit the specific needs of your skin. Solid skin is an aftereffect of predictable propensities so it is significant you follow a Facemask routine alongside a sound lifestyle.

www.ingramcontent.com/pod-product-compliance
Lightning Source LLC
Chambersburg PA
CBHW050251220526
45465CB00002B/640